HUMAN BODY COLORING BOOK FOR KIDS

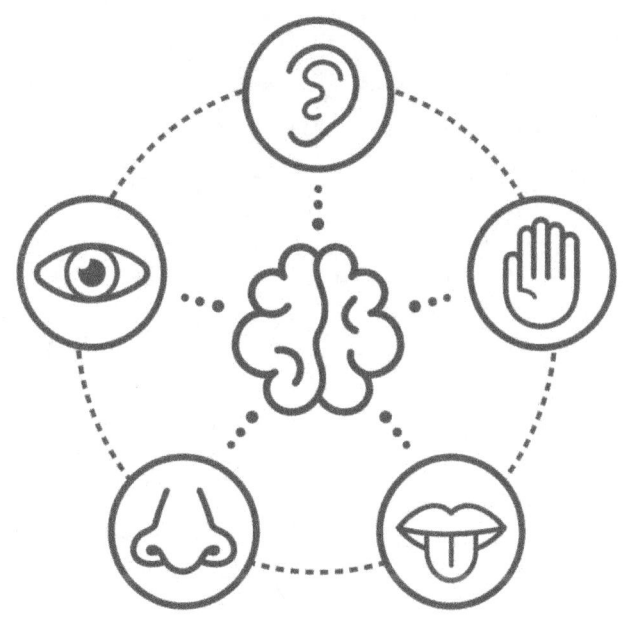

My First Human Body Parts and
Human Anatomy Coloring Book for Kids

HENRY DARWIN

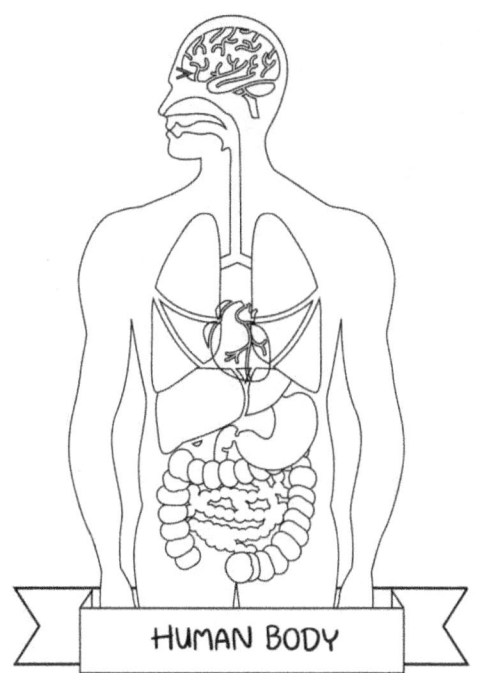

HUMAN BODY

Copyright © 2020 by Henry Darwin. All rights reserved.
No part of this book may be reproduced in any form or by any electronic or mechanical means, including information storage and retrieval systems, without written permission from the author, except for the use of brief quotations in a book review

BODY PART

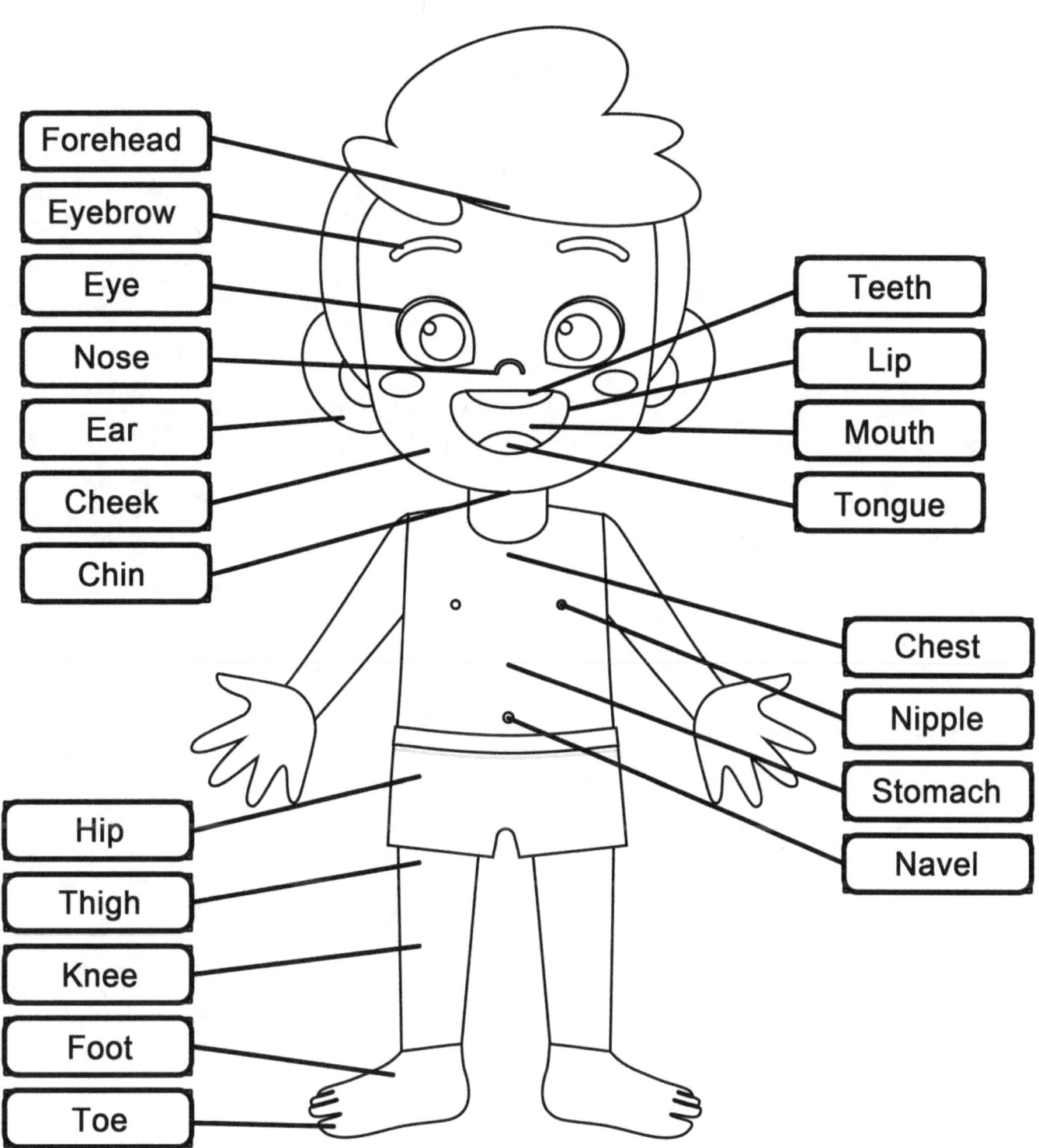

BODY PART

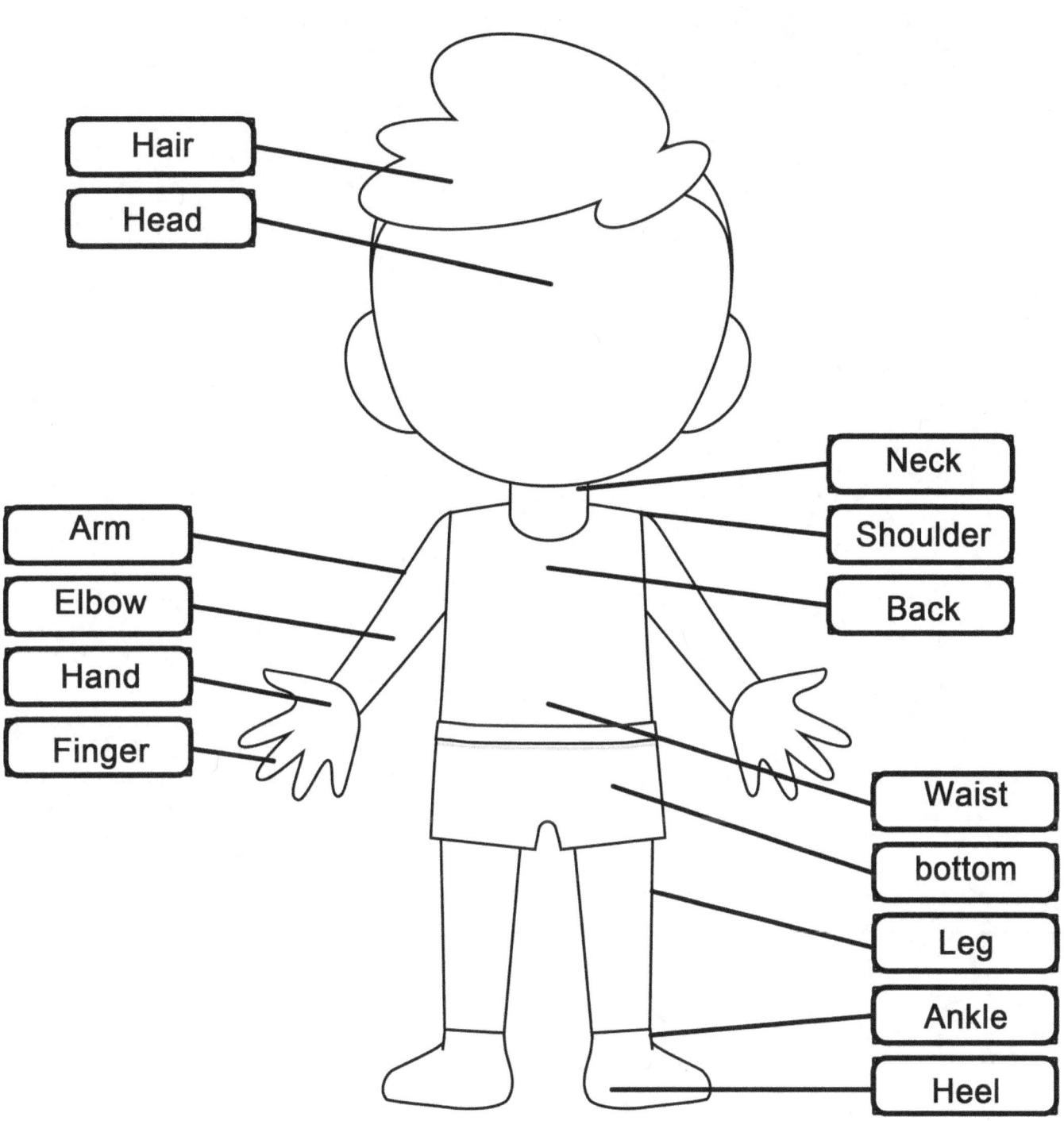

BODY PART

- HAIR
- EYEBROW
- NOSE
- LIP
- MOUTH
- TONGUE
- FOOT
- HEAD
- EYE
- EAR
- ARM
- HAND
- LEG

BODY ORGANS

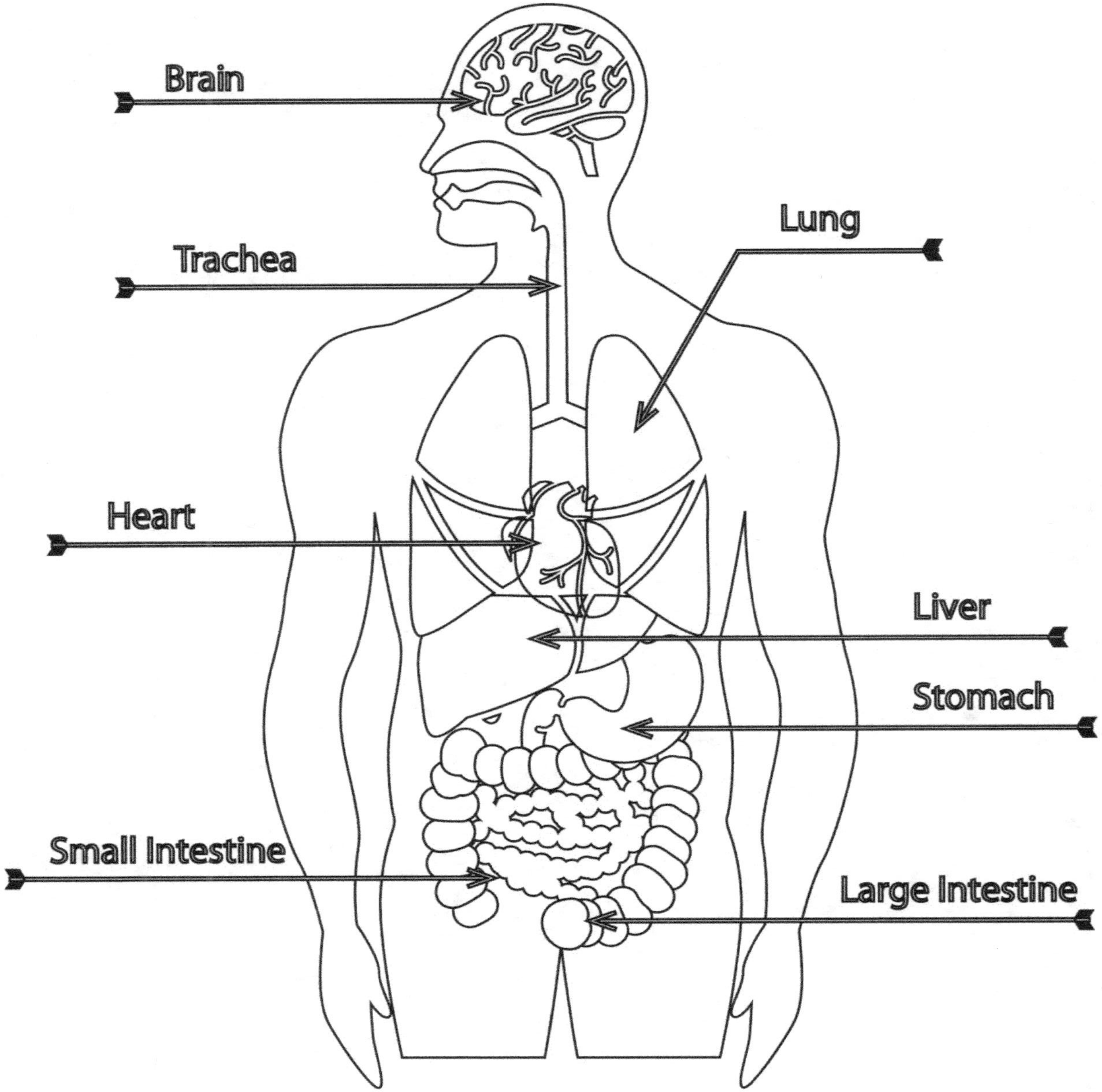

- Brain
- Lung
- Trachea
- Heart
- Liver
- Stomach
- Small Intestine
- Large Intestine

5 Senses

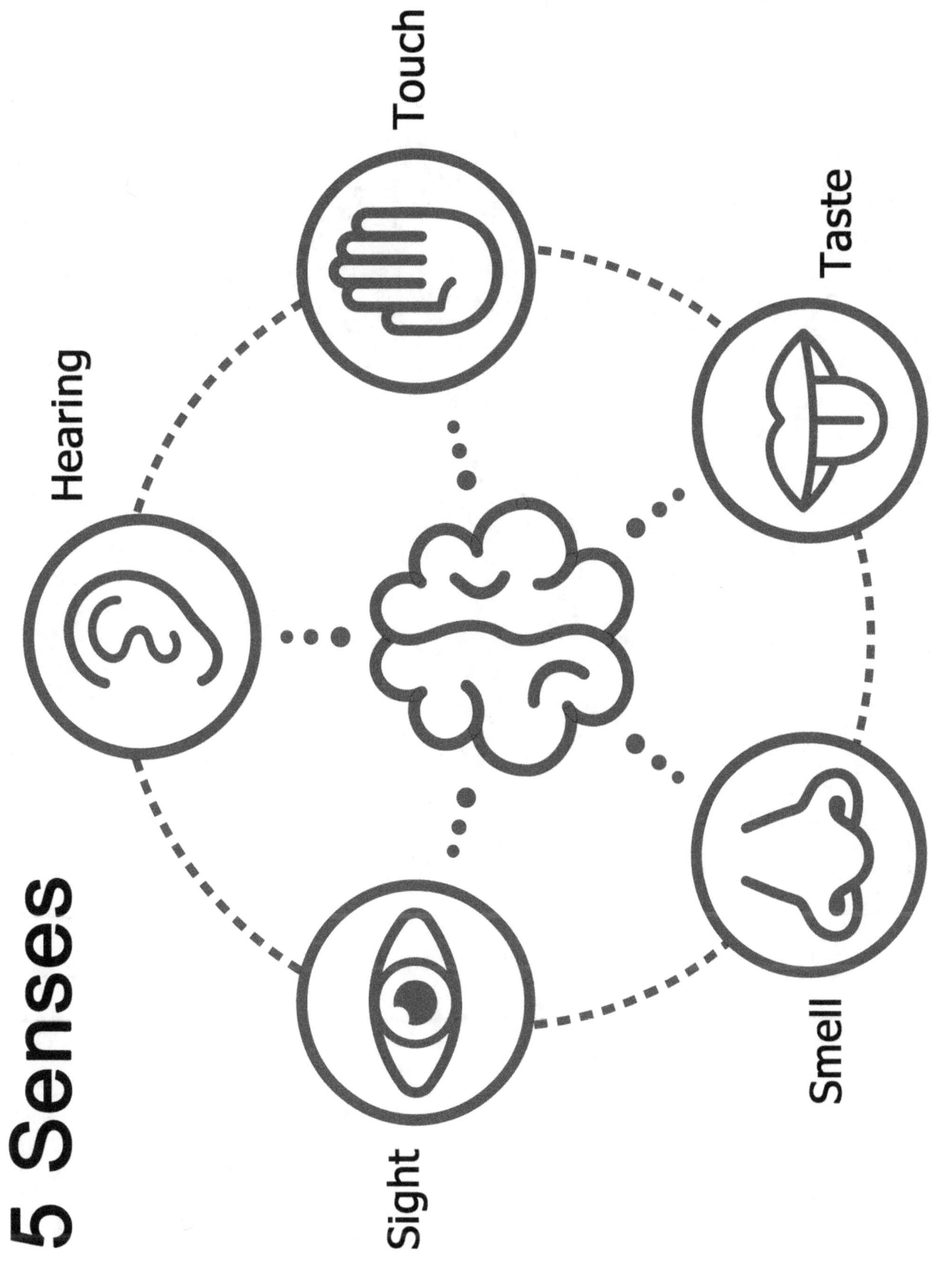

BRAIN

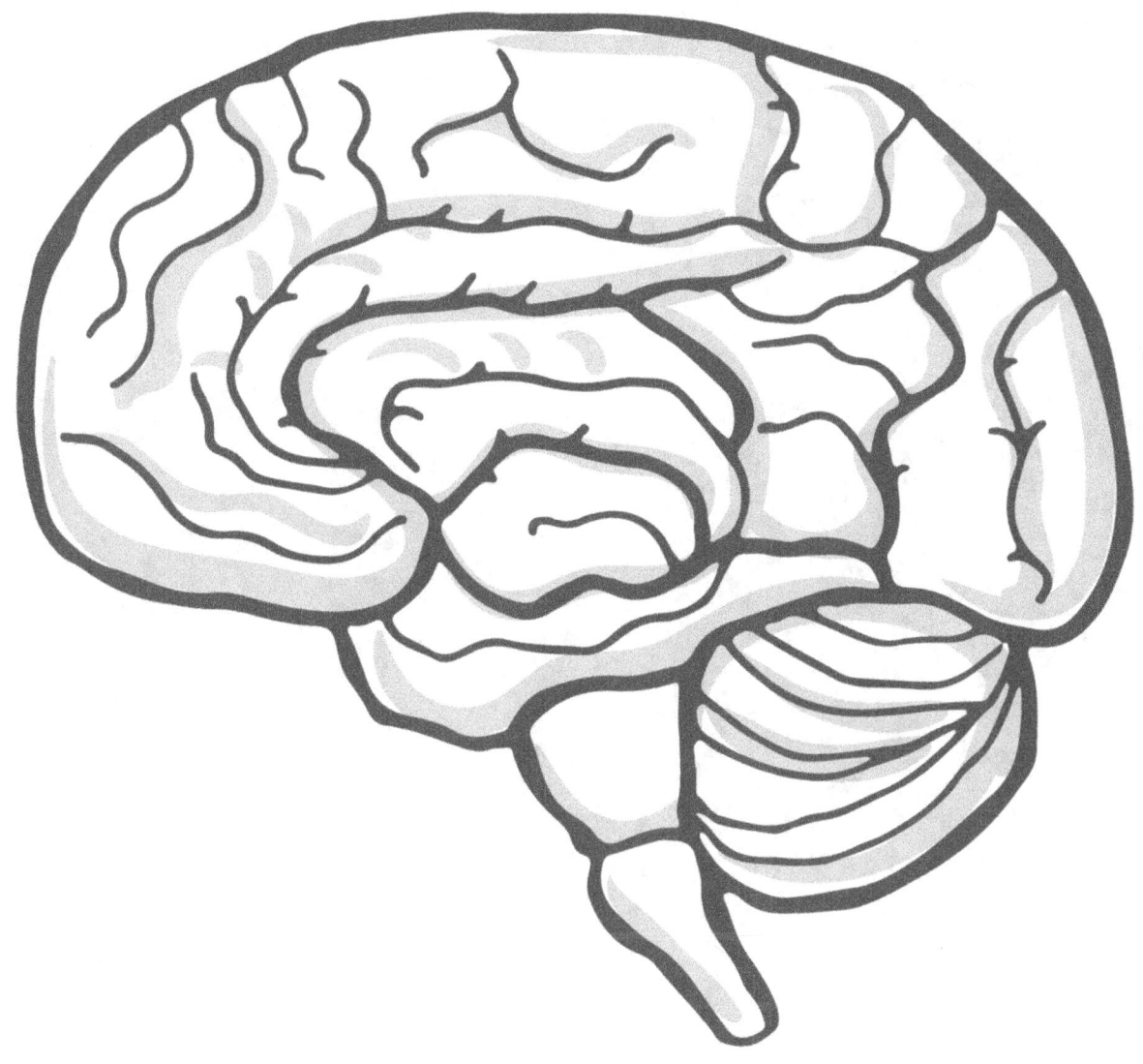

A brain is an organ that serves as the center of the nervous system in all human. It is located in the head. It is the most complex organ in a human body.

HEART

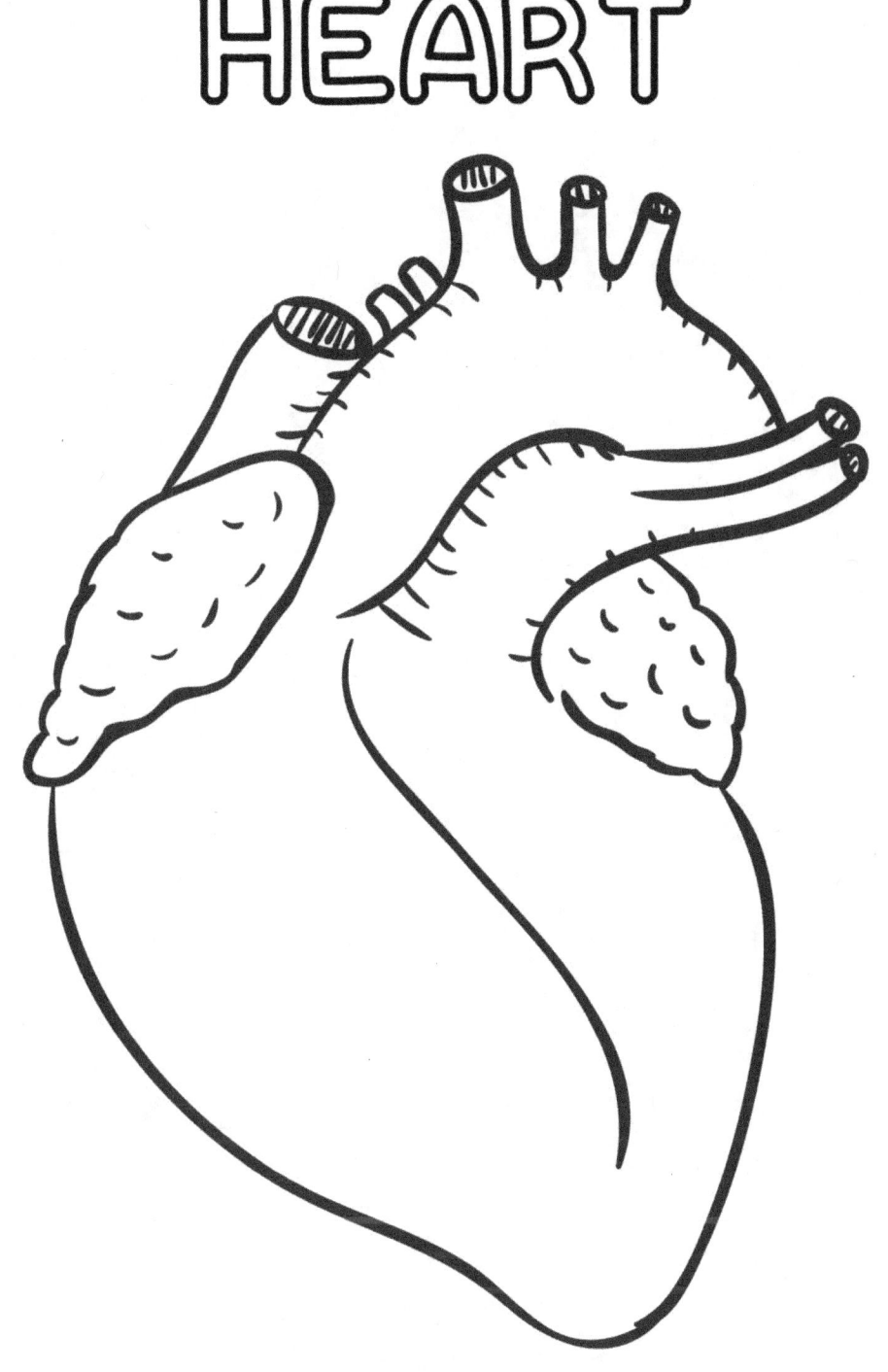

The heart is responsible for pumps blood through the blood vessels of the circulatory system. The pumped blood carries oxygen and nutrients to the body, while carrying metabolic waste such as carbon dioxide to the lungs. In humans, the heart is located between the lungs, in the middle compartment of the chest.

LIVER

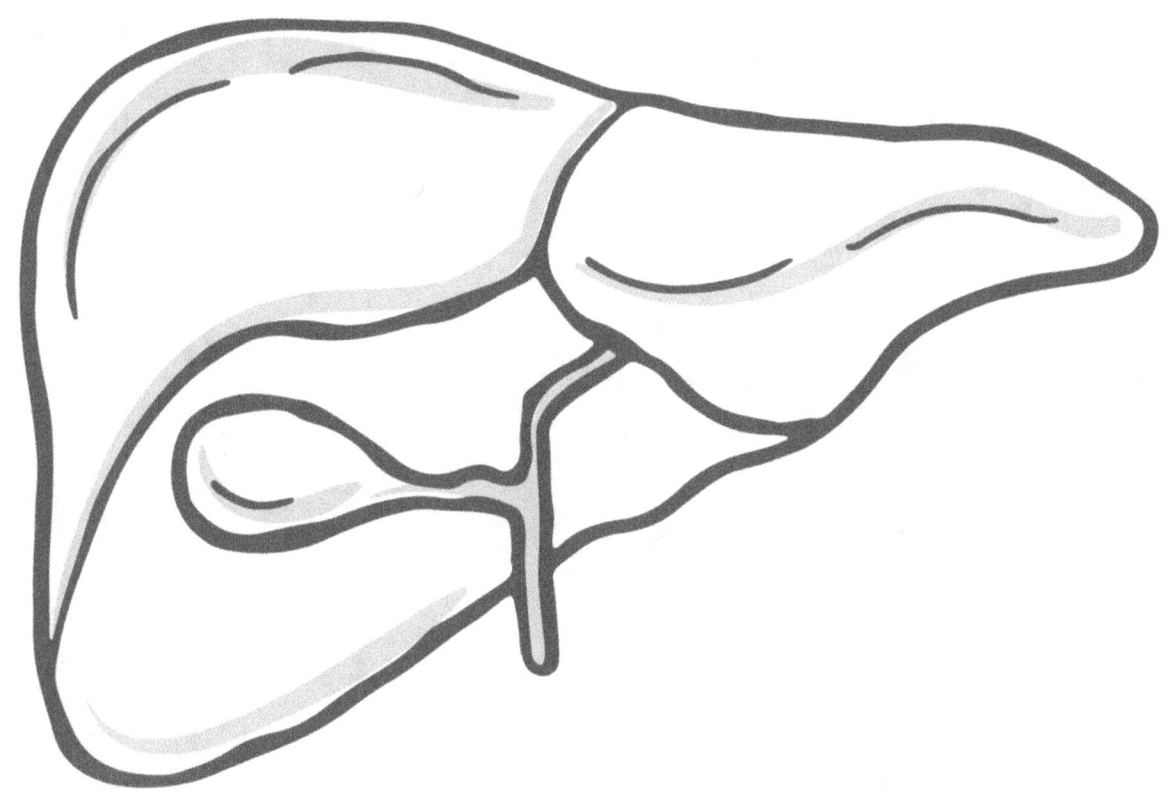

The liver is responsible for detoxifies various metabolites, synthesizes proteins and produces biochemicals necessary for digestion and growth. Its other roles in metabolism include the regulation of glycogen storage, decomposition of red blood cells, and the production of hormones.

KIDNEYS

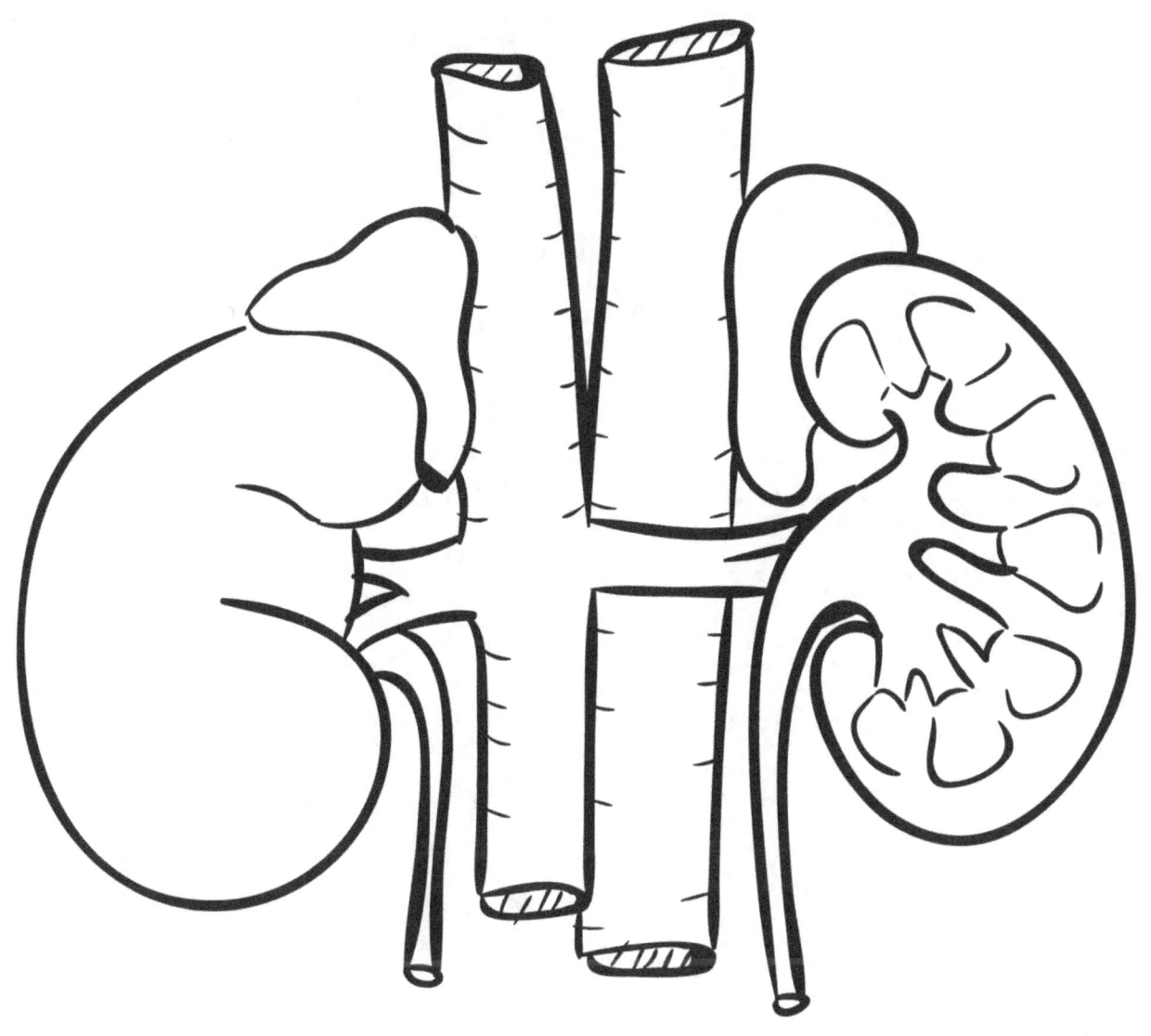

Kidneys is responsible for remove wastes and extra fluid from body into the urine. Kidneys also remove acid that is produced by the cells of body and maintain a healthy balance of water, salts, and minerals in blood.

LUNGS

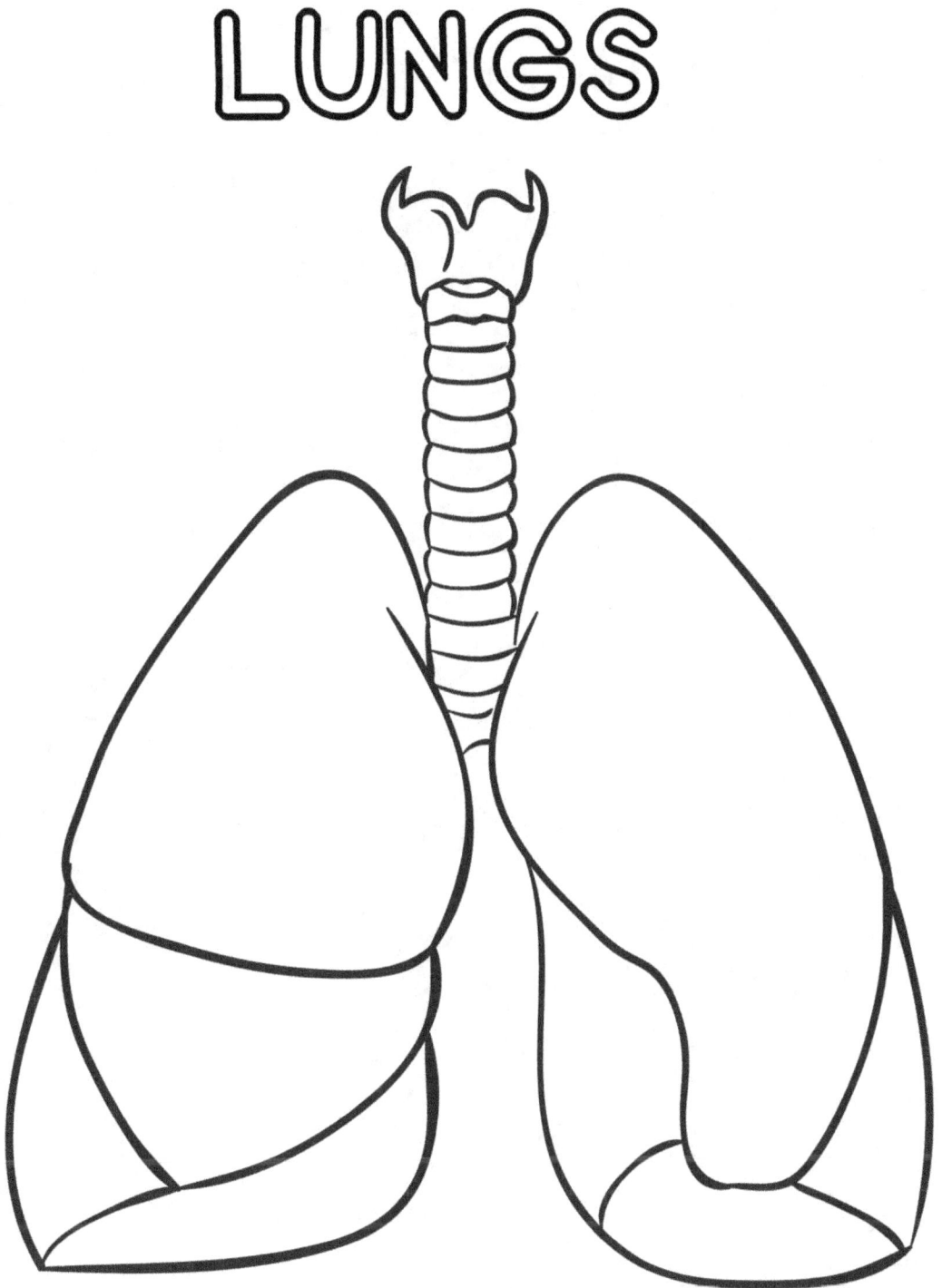

The lungs are the primary organs of the respiratory system in humans. The main function of the lungs is the process of gas exchange called respiration (or breathing).

INTESTINES

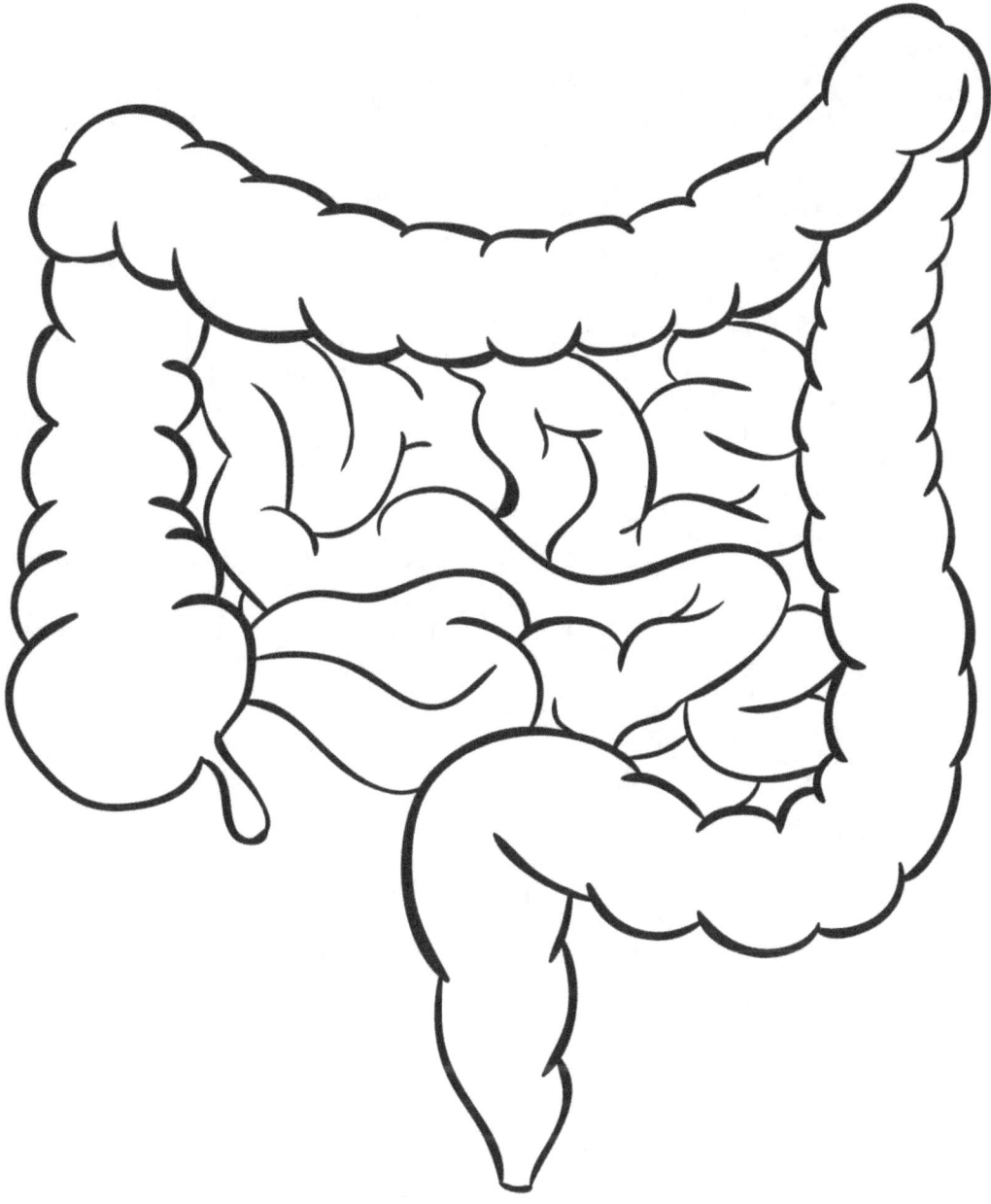

The intestines are a long, continuous tube running from the stomach to the anus. It's responsible for absorption of nutrients and water.
The intestines include the small intestine, large intestine, and rectum.
- *The small intestine* : responsible for absorb most of the nutrients from what we eat and drink.
- *The large intestine* : responsible for absorbs water from wastes, creating stool. Nerves there create the urge to defecate.

STOMACH

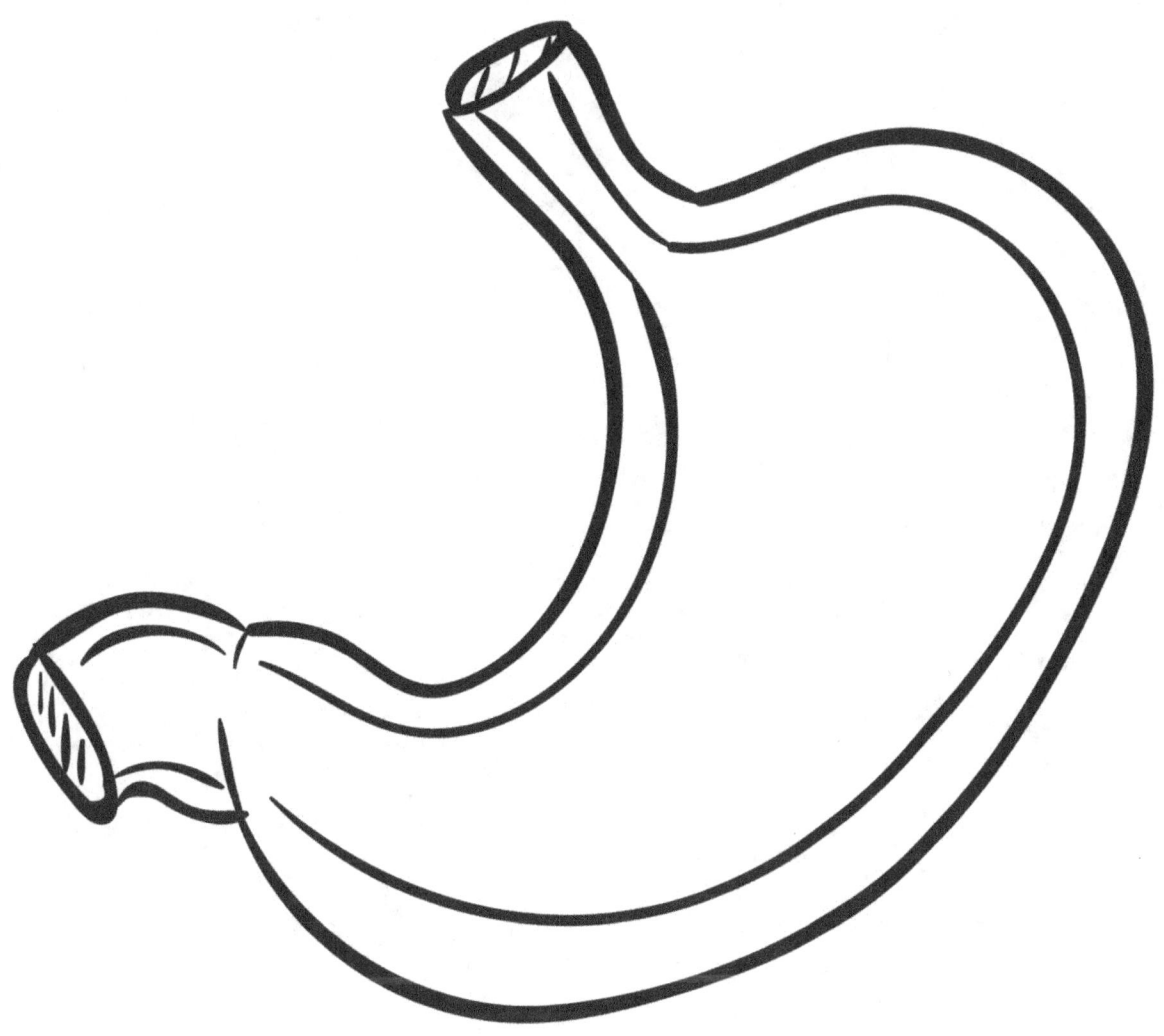

The stomach receives food from the esophagus. As food reaches the end of the esophagus, it enters the stomach. The stomach secretes acid and enzymes that digest food.

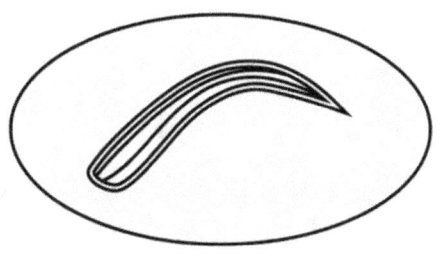
Eyebrow

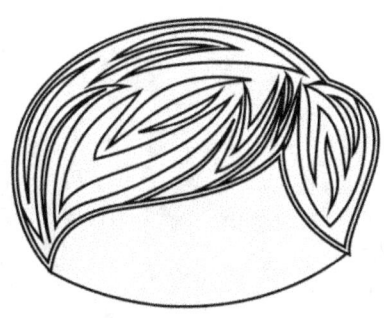
Hair

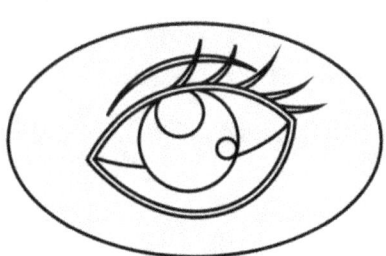
Eye

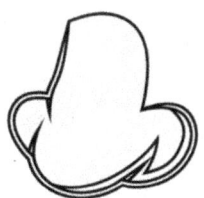
Nose

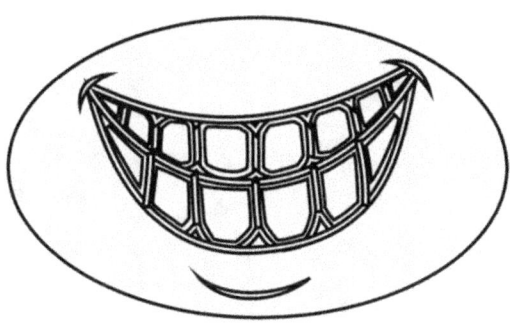
Teeth

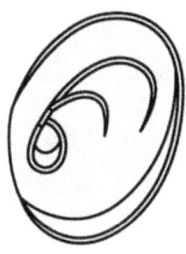
Ear

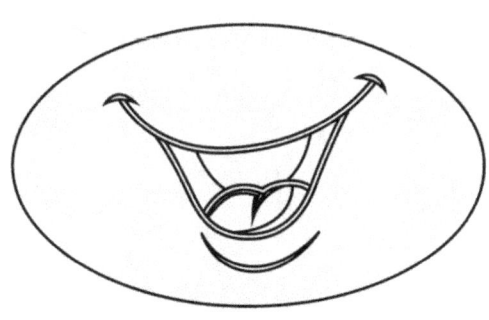
Mouth

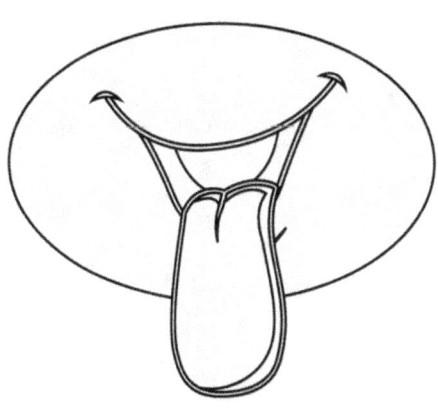
Tongue

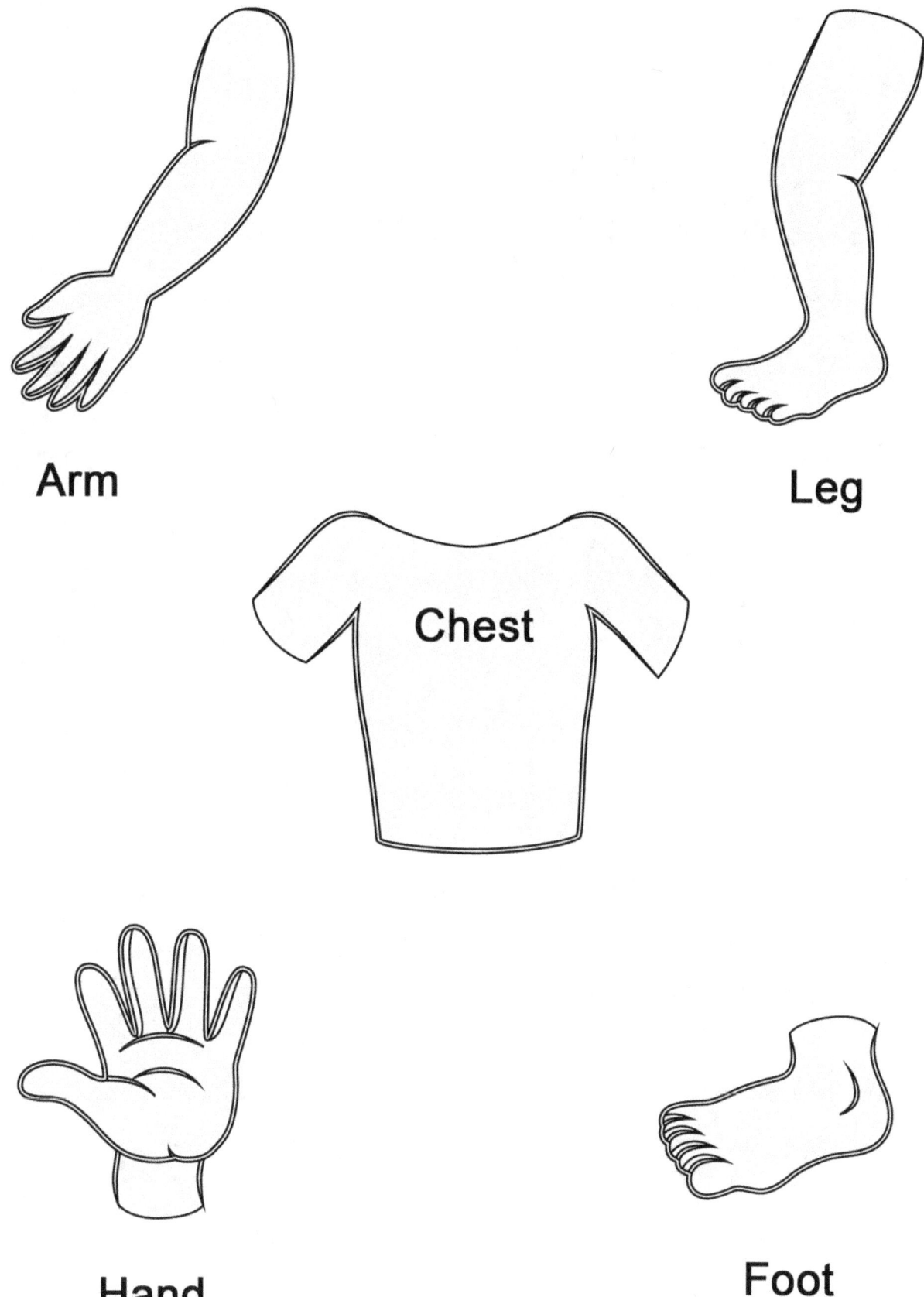

BODY PART

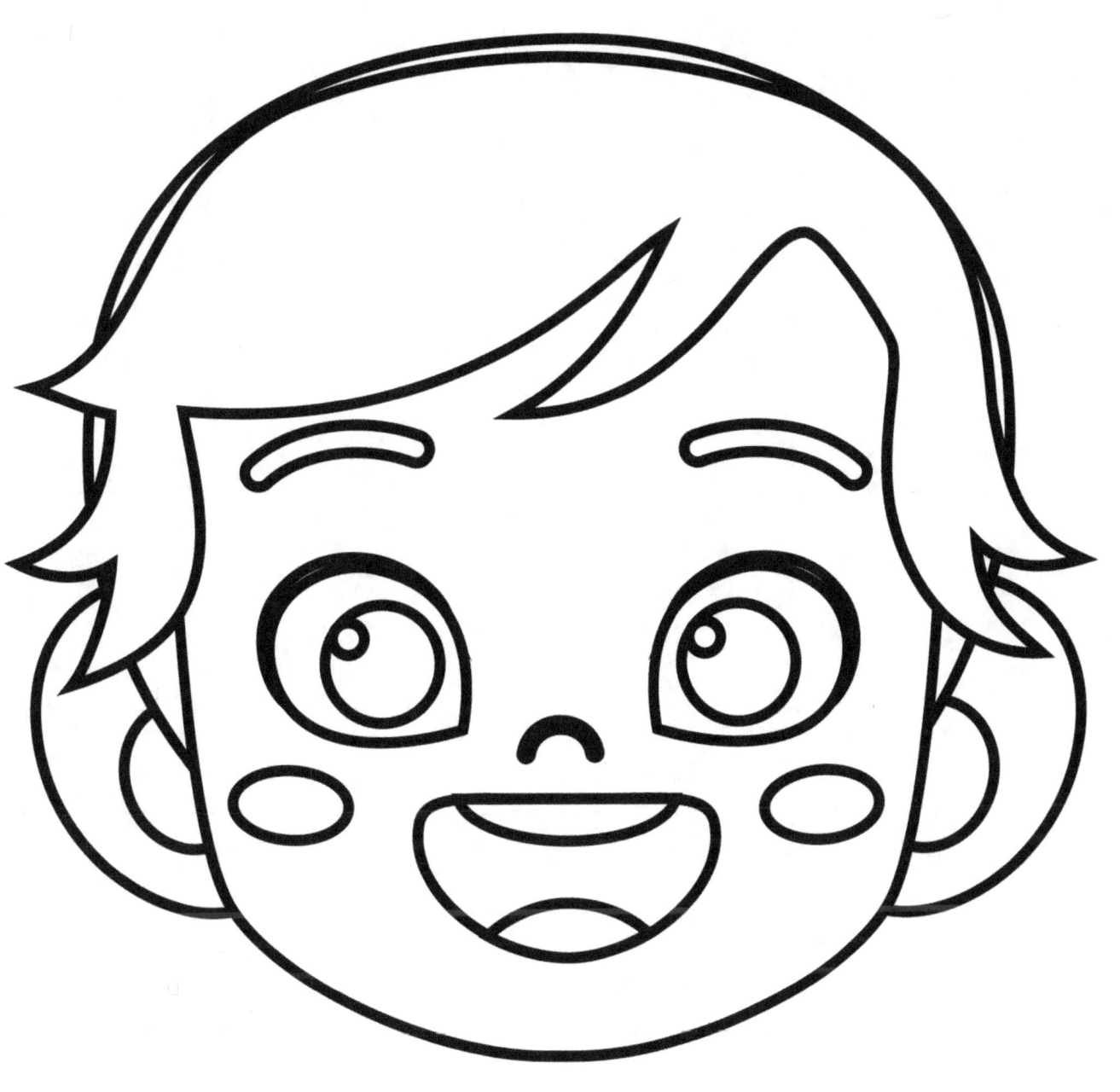

FACE

BODY PART

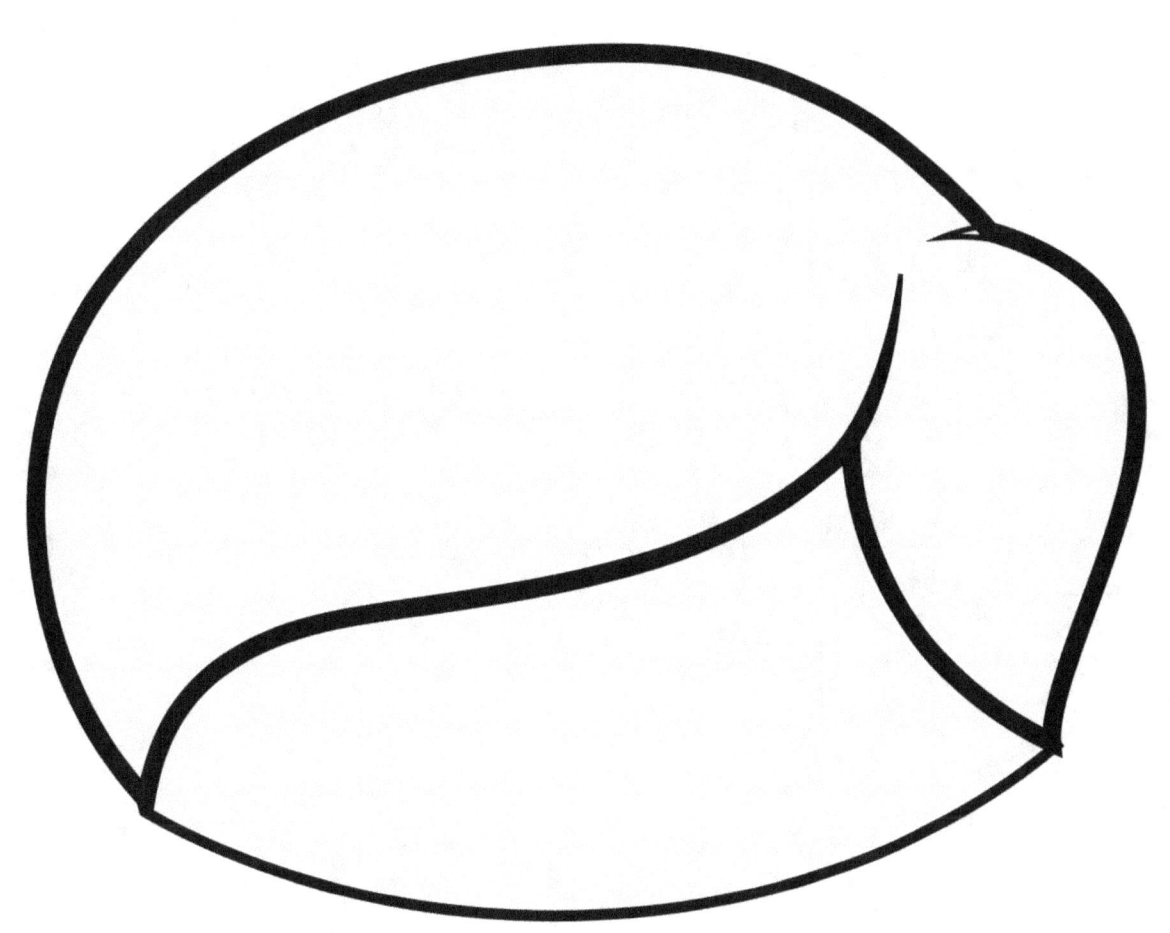

HAIR

BODY PART

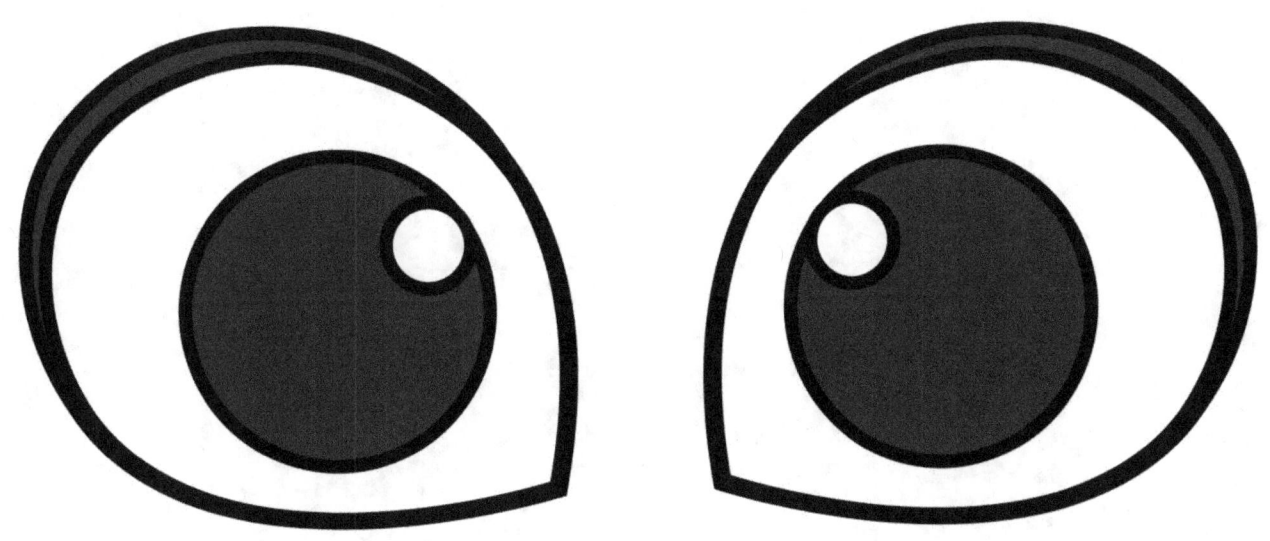

EYES

BODY PART

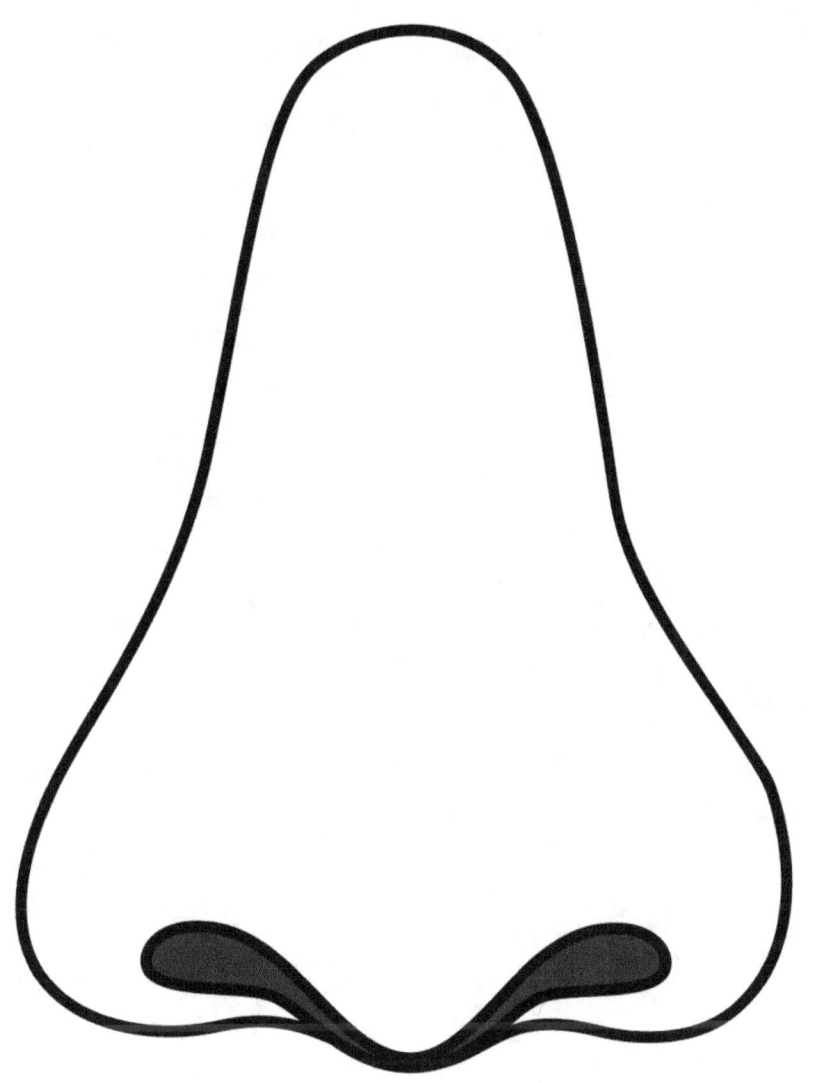

NOSE

BODY PART

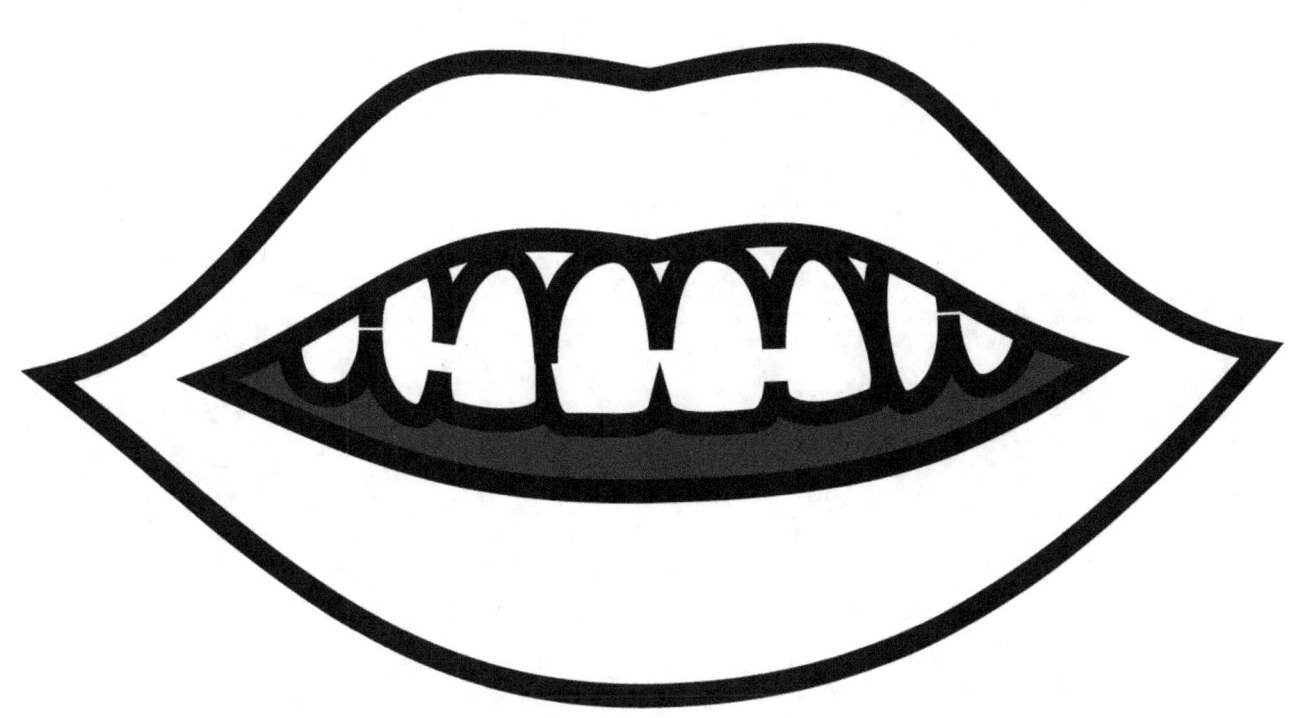

MOUTH

BODY PART

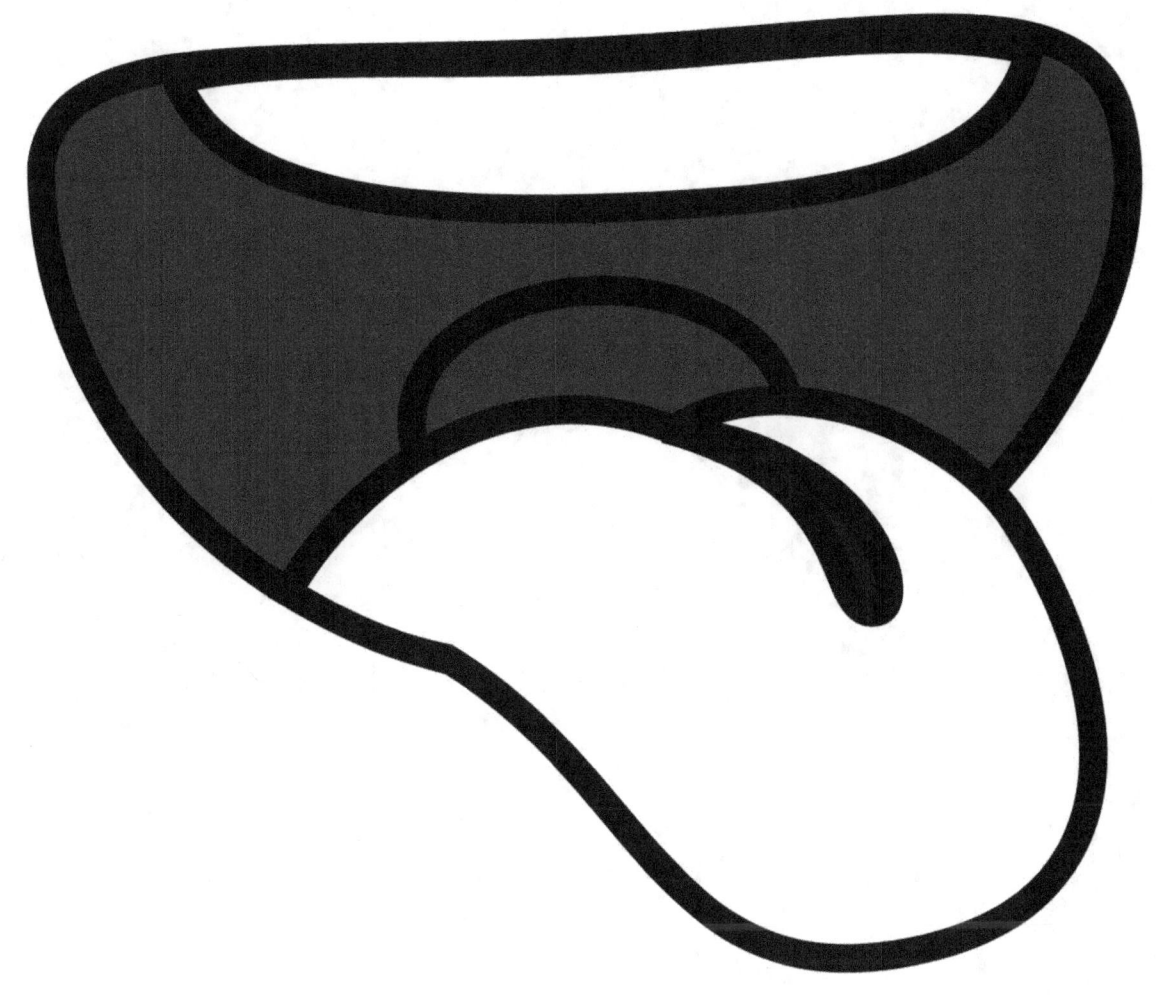

TONGUE

BODY PART

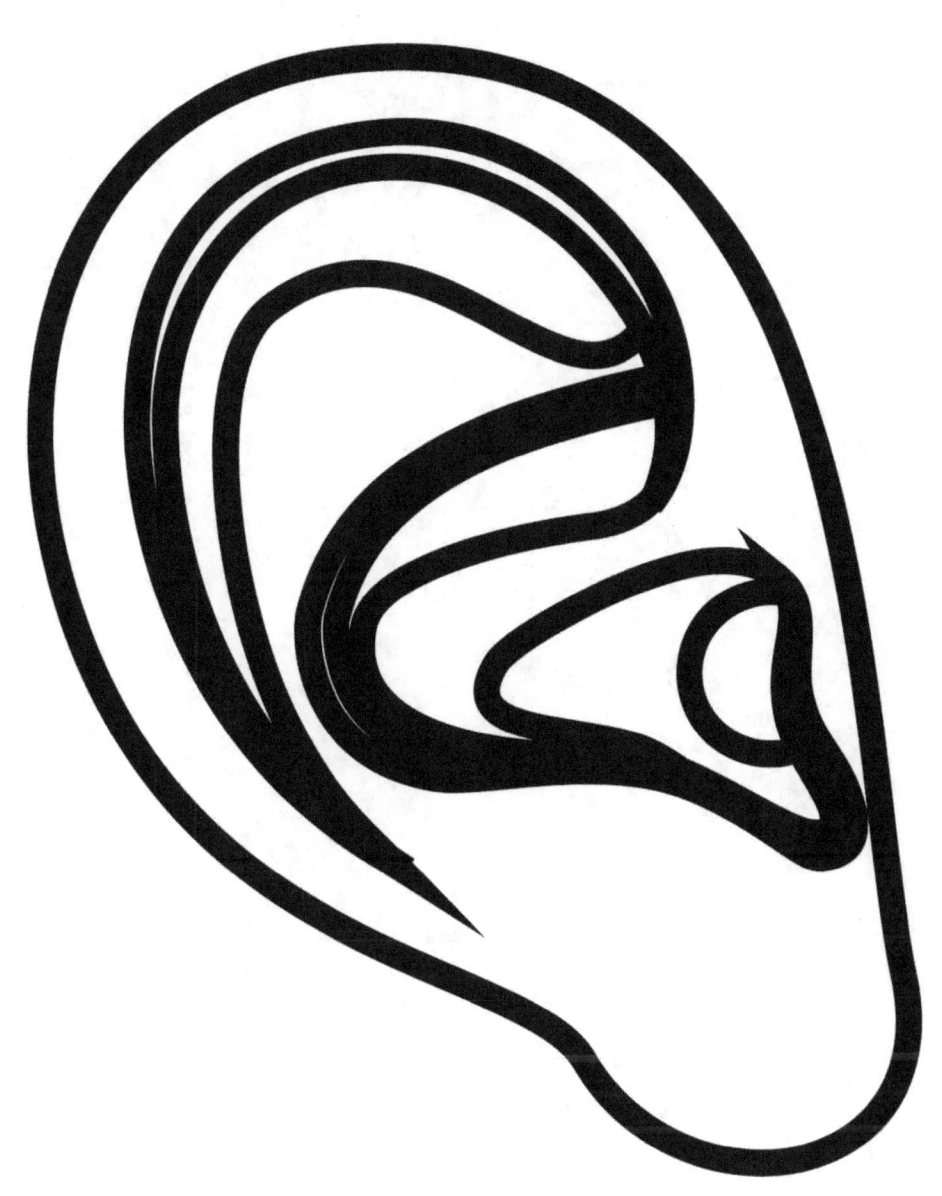

EAR

BODY PART

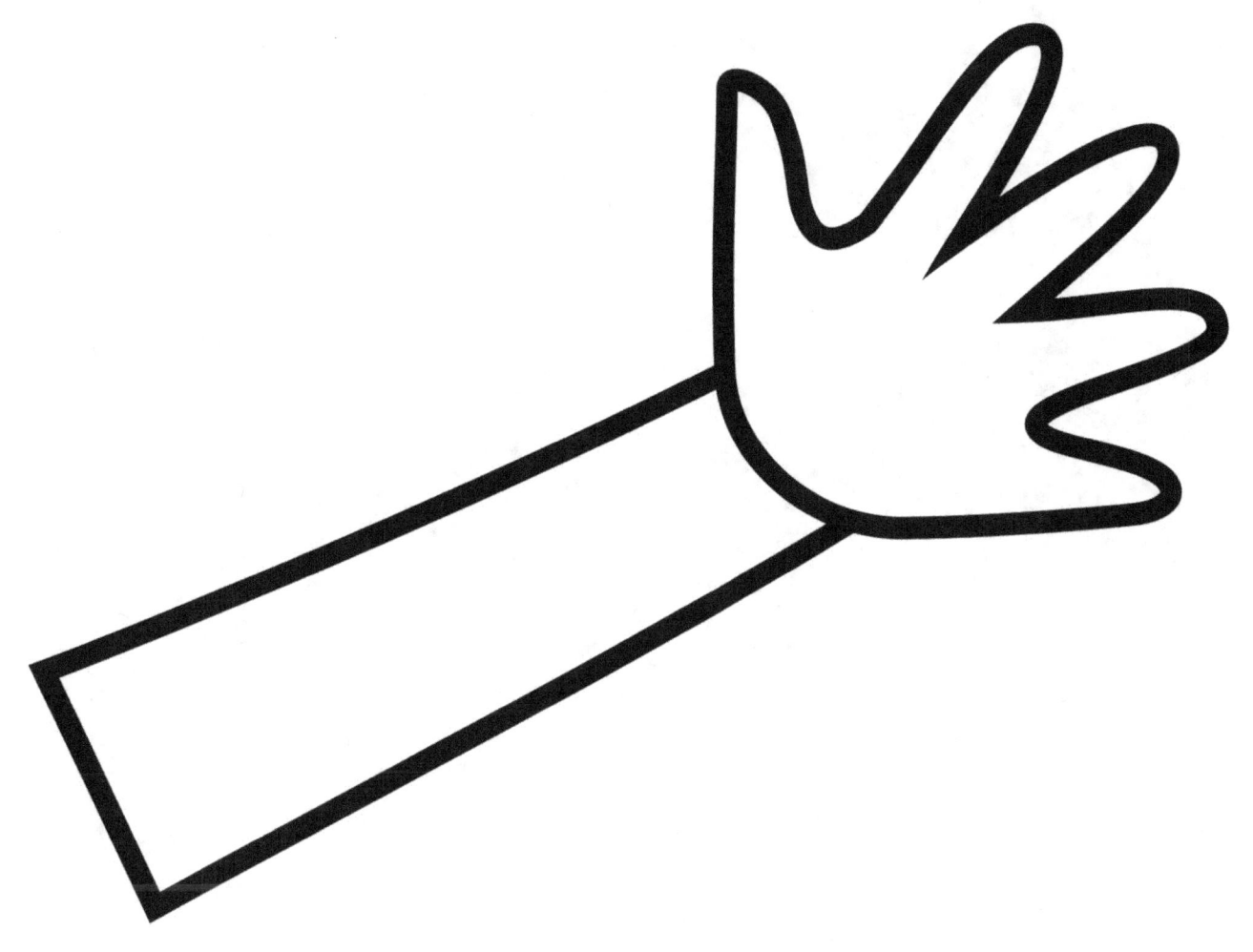

ARM

BODY PART

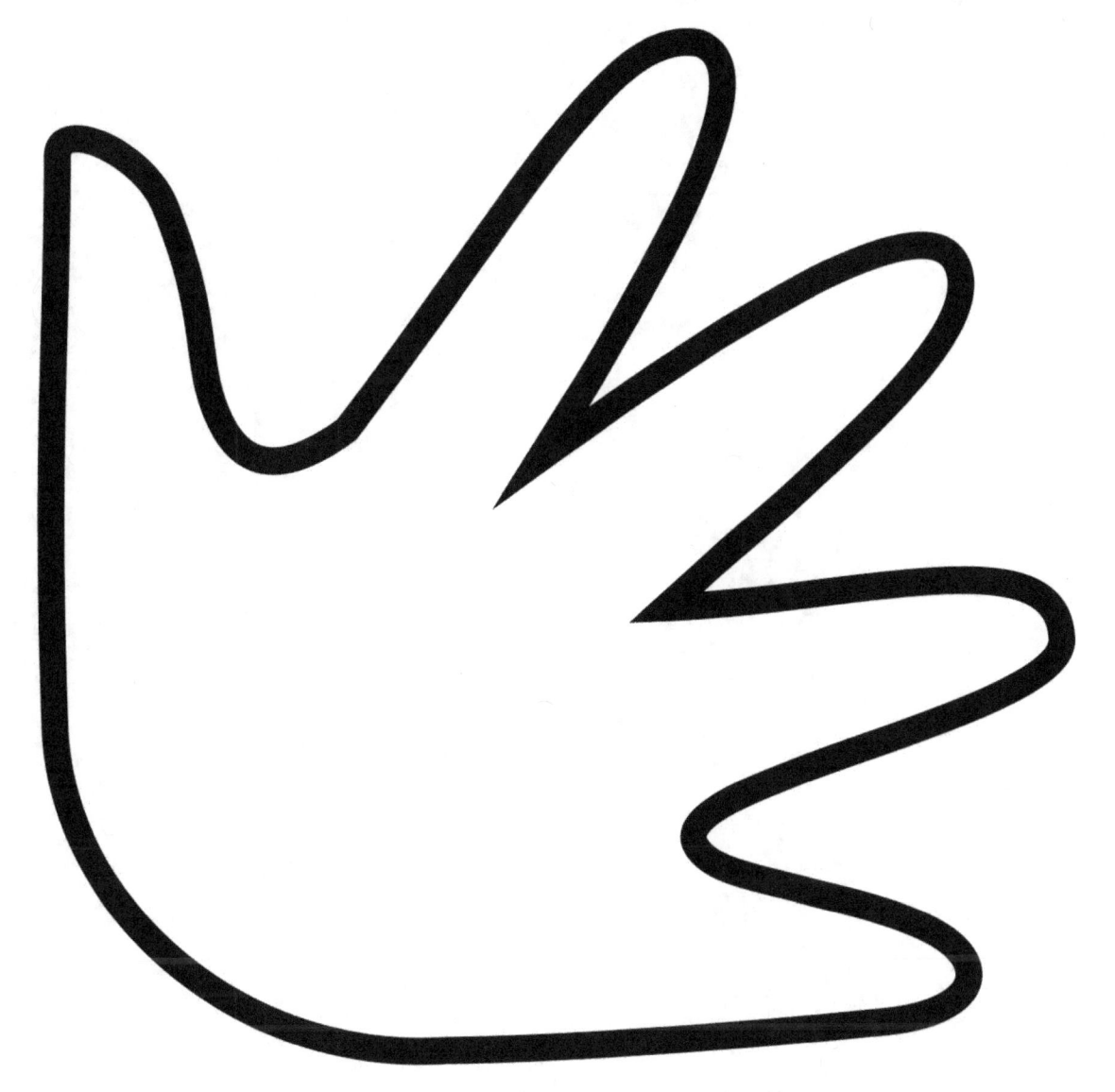

HAND

BODY PART

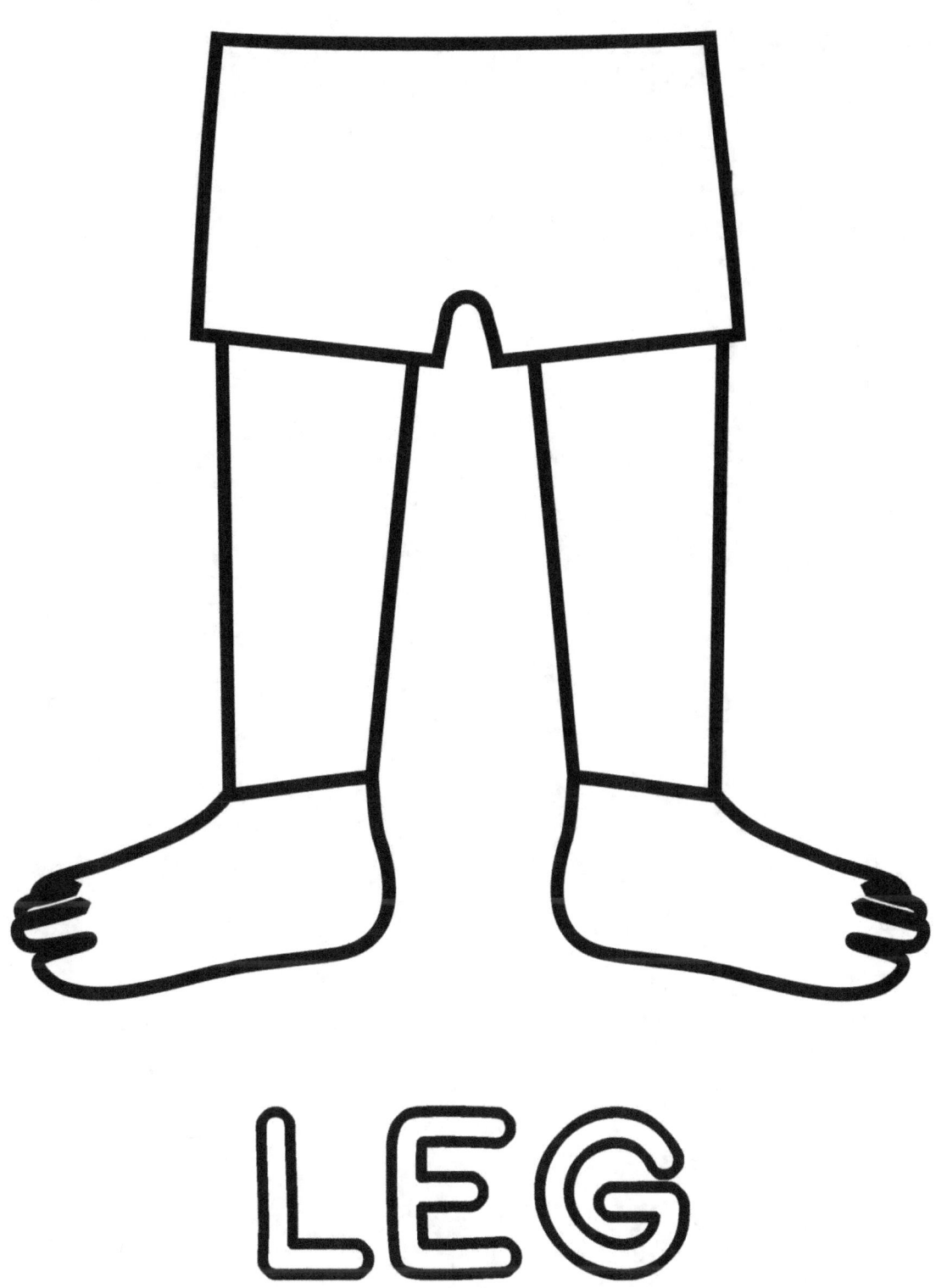

LEG

BODY PART

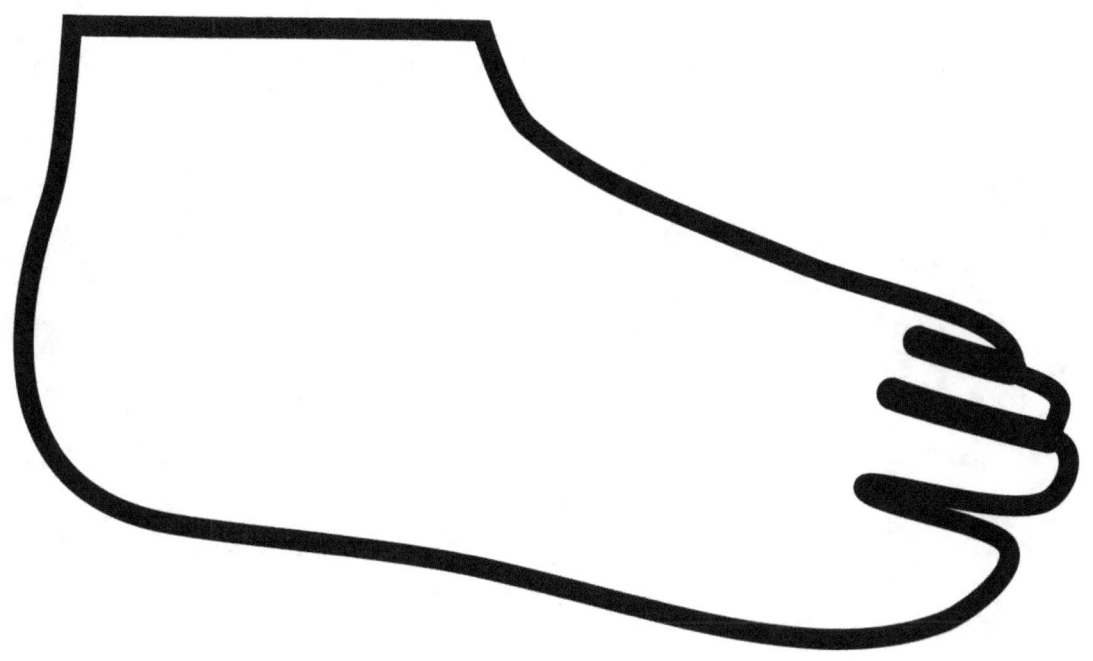

FOOT

www.ingramcontent.com/pod-product-compliance
Lightning Source LLC
Chambersburg PA
CBHW081528240526
45465CB00030B/3271